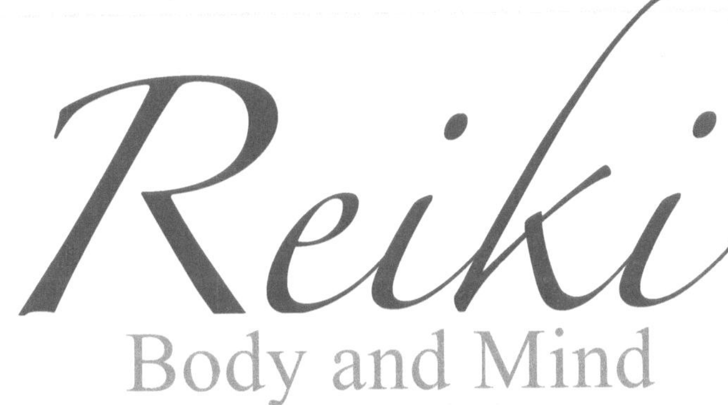

REIKI BODY AND MIND

Table Of Contents

The magic of Reiki can bring a few superb advantages into your life. With Reiki, you can decrease pressure, let go of passionate disturbance, and recuperate numerous ailments – both yours and those of others.

Be that as it may, you might be confounded by the immense measure of data accessible on this straightforward healing technique.

Additionally, new principles are continually being included from other recuperating systems, adding to the disarray.

In short, it is known that the first lessons of Dr. Mikao Usui, the Japanese educator and Shingon Buddhist minister who rediscovered this ancient system utilized by The Buddha.

The Origins of Reiki

Reiki has its underlying foundations in India. From that point it was passed to Tibet, China, and Japan. In the late nineteenth century, Dr. Mikao Usui, a Japanese specialist on a journey for otherworldly recuperating, happened upon a 1,100-year-old Buddhist original copy itemizing many healing strategies.

In perusing originally, Dr. Usui received a few practices from it to be utilized by anybody paying little respect to religion. The laying on of hands depicted in that, he marked 'Reiki' (Universal Life Force Energy).

Essentially, we're composed of energy. Attunement or empowerment through a Reiki Master enables us to recharge ourselves with this Universal Life Force Energy, which is everywhere.

"When you heal yourself and assist others with their self-healing,

you heal the Earth. You do make a difference." – Laurel Steinhice

Dissolving Emotional Blocks and Healing the Body

On the enthusiastic dimension, Reiki recuperates by dissolving the blocks we make through our negative decisions and contemplations. This "stuck" energy as often as possible shows up as ailment in the body.

For instance, blockages can show as ulcers, cerebral pains or stomach pains. Unexpressed displeasure and sadness can cause tumors, while controlling attitudes of mind can prompt rheumatoid joint inflammation.

An Intelligent Energy

A stunning aspect concerning Reiki is that it's an astute vitality and knows which zones of the body need healing. So in the event that you place your hands on an individual's head to heal a cerebral pain, the vitality from your hands will likewise go to different spots where it's required in that individual's body.

Reiki for Emotional and Mental Balance

Reiki is exceptionally compelling for enthusiastic and mental equalization. Customary self treatments will guarantee that you don't actually get worried. What's more, with mental equalization comes better memory and clarity.

A decent Reiki healer can tell what enthusiastic difficulties you have and help you to heal them. For example, a healer can call attention to negative idea patterns with the goal that you can change your state of mind. Instinct is additionally improved with the act of Reiki.

"Our sorrows and wounds are healed only when we touch them with compassion." – The Buddha

Reiki and Animals: A Strange Effect of Reiki

A Reiki professional is a channel of the Universal Life Force. Thusly, he can't state that he has recuperated somebody. Individuals must be available to the treatment regardless of whether they're on the wary side. Being open enables their bodies to intuitively draw the vitality required.

Numerous specialists find that creatures are more open to the vitality than people. Creatures don't have questions.

Jack, a Reiki professional, has a puppy that rejects his Reiki treatments. He says: "It's bizarre. At the point when my puppy has a belly ache, I lay my hands on her stomach yet she generally endeavors to move away. Furthermore, I thought creatures have no blockages."

While all in all, creatures are progressively open to Reiki, some don't care for it. Maybe they're ready to feel the energy all the more intensely. On the off chance that they're genuinely sick, they may have their own arrangements about their change and don't need anything to meddle.

Frequently, in instances of a terminal disease, creatures realize it's their opportunity to pass on. The Reiki can't stop that. Along these lines, a healer must know how wiped out the creature is before he endeavors to recuperate.

Nonetheless, paying little heed to whether the creature acknowledges recuperating or not, your demonstration of benevolence is a commitment toward the healing of the planet.

At the point when a creature is in intense torment, it might be anxious amid the initial couple of minutes when you start healing in light of the fact that Reiki will in general strengthen the torment. On the off chance that the creature protests here and there, drift your hands over the creature as opposed to contacting it specifically or place your hands delicately on the animal while you converse with it soothingly.

In the event that you've been started into second degree Reiki, you can utilize the Sei Hei Kei image to initially quiet the creature. Or on the other hand as Dr. Hartman, a veterinarian, recommends in The Reiki Handbook, by Larry Arnold and Sandy Nevius, you can start at the crown position. This has a quieting impact on canines and felines.

Hartman includes that for back wounds it's great to put the fingers pointing down the spine. Additionally, a few creatures might be too panicked to even consider facing you. In such cases, you can approach them looking indistinguishable way from they are, so they can't see you, and can just feel your hands.

A second degree Reiki expert, Hartman has made them flabbergast healing encounters with creatures. In one example, he spared a fundamentally sick puppy from death with two hours of persistent Reiki. He says there are numerous contrasts between treating creatures and treating people.

One of the imperative contrasts is as to the pacing of treatments. People at first require four sequential long periods of treatment pursued by maybe three sessions per week. Be that as it may, creatures by and large need successive long stretches of healing until they demonstrate increased improvement.

"In a world older and more complete than ours they move

finished and complete, gifted with extensions of the

senses we have lost or never attained, living by voices we

shall never hear. They are not brethren, they are not underlings;

they are other nations, caught with ourselves in the net of life

and time, fellow prisoners of the splendor and

travail of the earth." – Henry Beston

Animals and Reiki: Another Example

Darline has a cluster of donkeys on her farm. When one of them fundamentally harmed a rear leg, breaking the bone, the appendage created gangrene. The vet's decision was to "put the creature down" as nothing should be possible about the leg and the gangrene was spreading.

In any case, Darline wouldn't know about it. She requested two or three weeks' time, amid which she would send removed Reiki treatments to the creature and complete a hands-on recuperating at whatever point conceivable.

After only two hands-on healings and 12 days of day by day far off treatment, every session enduring 15 minutes, the bones became back, the gangrene disappeared, and the donkey started to run utilizing the leg. As a reward, he wound up friendlier. He wound up more settled, and promptly permitted Darline to heal him.

Strikingly, a couple of months after her Darline's Reiki commencement, she saw that the focuses of her palms tingled. The left palm built up a particular dip in the middle. She saw a similar sign in the palm of another lady who was a confidence healer and had additionally restored some serious ailments.

Beguiled, Darline consulted a Reiki Master, who advised her there was a vortex of energy issuing from the focal point of her palms. The palm "chakras" had opened up.

The dip in her left palm remains. And when she's near someone seriously ill, her palms get hot.

"With all beings and all things we shall be relatives."

– Sioux Indian precept

How to Choose Your Reiki Master

Look for a master in the heredity of Dr. Usui. Along these lines you'll realize that you're getting the first attunement portrayed in the Buddhist original manuscript he found, The Tantra of the Lightning Flash That Heals the Body and Illumines the Mind.

Finding a self-acknowledged master is incredibly troublesome, however don't stress a lot over it. The ace is just the channel for the attunement. The power dwells in the attunement itself.

Be that as it may, do search for an euphoric master who isn't pleased about his healings. All things considered, he is just a channel for the recuperating energy.

A decent Reiki master won't push his understudies to do second and third degree Reiki after the underlying commencement is finished. The understudy must feel prepared for the following dimension after adequate practice. The master ought to have something like three years of experience on the way.

Keep in mind that there's no such thing as a "great master" in spite of the fact that there are some who allude to themselves along these lines. This just mirrors their hunger for power and status.

One of the reasons for the development of "grand masters" is the fact that the third degree, originally was determined for those who want to attune others, was split into two levels - one for the spiritual boost provided to holders of the second degree through the receipt of the "master symbol," and the other for teaching the attunement. This was of course only a money-making ploy.

It's smarter to avoid types of Reiki that utilization dream images made by different individuals.

Here are four hotspots for attunements that are genuine:

+ Customary Reiki through Usui and his understudies Hayashi, Takata, and Takata's 22 understudies (if they educate Reiki in its fundamental structure and keep the transmission unadulterated).

+ Heredities followed back to Usui through Hayashi and his understudy, the Zen priest, Sensei Takeuchi.

✦ Men Chhos Rei Kei International, in view of Dr.

Usui's notes and the sutra that enlivened him.

✦ Usui Reiki Ryobo Gakkei, the customary Reiki

rehearsed in Japan in a solid genealogy.

The First Degree

What's it like to study Reiki? The First Degree is given in a progression of four attunements. There must be a gap of 24 hours between the second and third attunement.

The attunements can occur over a four-day or two-day time frame. You'll need to commit the whole day, so guarantee you've disappeared from office and family obligations.

At each dimension, your body needs 21 days to completely soak up the attunements. After the primary degree, you should rehearse on yourself and on others for at least three months before proceeding onward to the second degree.

The attunement is an excellent, delicate custom amid which the master contacts your palms and the bottoms of your feet and tenderly blows on them.

In any case, the attunement doesn't give you anything you didn't have previously. It just opens you up to a greater amount of the general life drive.

Starting here on, Reiki will stream out of your hands and feet the moment you plan to heal. Amid the 21 days of purifying after your first degree, your body will alter itself to the new vitality and your atmosphere and chakras will clear. You ought to complete a day by day self healing amid this period.

Darline says that the main time she could really feel the sap ascending in a plant was after her First Degree amid the purging and practice period. "It resembled power," she says. "I unquestionably made my papaya tree develop tall and solid actually quick with the Reiki. It gave me a wealth of fine natural product."

"The only work that will ultimately bring any good to any of us is

the work of contributing to the healing of the world."

– Marianne Williamson

The Second Degree

This dimension involves only one attunement. You are given three images that empower Reiki to rise above existence. Now, you can heal others through "inaccessible healing."

Second Degree experts are urged to heal themselves on a psychological and passionate dimension, so past damages fall far from them. It's conceivable to get through conduct and thought designs identified with the insurance of your conscience.

Don't Expect Reiki to Fix Everything

Vicki, a second degree professional, says, "I don't know you can heal emotional and mental injuries with Reiki. I don't assume I had the capacity to dispose of the blockages, that my tragic adolescence made in me. I don't consider my youth, however I realize it influences me somehow or another.

I even influenced my significant other and youthful child to experience the main degree attunements, however that did not spare my marriage. My better half had an issue with liquor and I thought Reiki would help fix him however he wasn't prepared. My Reiki couldn't shield me from his maltreatment, yet it made me feel more quiet."

Vicky was inevitably ready to free herself from her marriage, however it wasn't through Reiki. The fact of the matter is that one must not expect the outlandish from Reiki.

So What Can You Expect From Reiki?

You can positively hope to most likely channel healings on a physical dimension. You can quiet personalities and help recuperate infections and affliction.

Discharging pressure and strain and mitigating the brain is the most imperative nature of Reiki, as indicated by Dr. Usui. Restorative specialists state that disposing of pressure, which harms the insusceptible framework, counteracts numerous diseases.

With Reiki, you can likewise help the vitality of plants, invigorate the water you drink, recuperate creatures, and the sky is the limit from there. Some even charge dead batteries with Reiki.

Notwithstanding, don't guarantee your patients that you can fix their disease with Reiki or get a particular outcomes. As Diane Stein says in her fantastic book, Essential Reiki:

> "The healer can only promise that Reiki benefits everyone that experiences it . . . Reiki relieves pain, speeds the healing process, stops bleeding, relaxes the receiver and balances the person's chakras and aura energy. Respiration

slows during a Reiki session and blood

pressure lowers; emotional calming occurs."

Ultimately, Reiki is beneficial. However, Reiki itself

knows in what way to benefit an individual. As a healer,

you will want to focus on your intention and release

attachment to results.

"Healing may not be so much about getting better,

as about

letting go of everything that isn't you - all of the

expectations,

all of the beliefs - and becoming who you are."

– Rachel Naomi Remen

Preparing For a Treatment

Before you give a treatment, here are a few hints to guarantee that your space is ideally set okay with healing:

Make a calm, agreeable, and mitigating condition.

Give a light cover or sheet and a container of tissues for your patient within simple reach.

Have your patient remove his glasses, coat, shoes, belt, vest, tie, scarf, and gems worn around the neck. A few people will likewise need to remove any gems that encloses the body, for example, rings or arm ornaments.

The apparel ought not be excessively tight - no supports or pantyhose.

Request that your patient rests and spot a pad underneath the head and furthermore under the knees.

See whether there's been any real medical procedure, damage, or sicknesses.

Guarantee the patient's feet are not crossed.

Wash your hands before you start. Keep your fingers together amid the healing.

Give the entire body treatment (constantly done except if it's a crisis circumstance) before you center around treating the affliction.

A few experts are sufficiently blessed to have a space committed to Reiki. In the event that you are a back rub specialist or substantial healer, this might be the situation for you. In any case, it's absolutely a bit much. Numerous profoundly successful treatments have been given on somebody's lounge room floor!

Amid Treatment

Your patient will feel heat from your hands. In some cases they'll encounter extreme warmth, despite the fact that it isn't hurtful to the skin. Reiki warmth can be felt through throws and attire. For the most part, the warmth will increment as per the seriousness of the sickness.

Here and there, an individual can feel warmth from the healer's hands notwithstanding when he's not being contacted specifically. What's more, in some cases you may find that Reiki puts a patient to rest. In the event that this occurs, let the individual rest. It will support the healing procedure.

> "To heal from the inside out is the key."
>
> - Wynonna Judd

You Are Healed When You Heal

This is a superb aspect regarding Reiki. When you heal somebody, you receive a recuperating consequently. You'll never feel drained or exhausted after a healing session since you're utilizing general life vitality, not your own.

Since Reiki has worked in insurance, you don't assume the disease or state of the one you heal.

Health: A Matter of Balance

It's your duty to tell those you recuperate that most infirmities are appearances of inward unsettling influences and they ought to dig profound inside themselves to find the reason. On the off chance that they're quiet and adjusted, they can regularly evade sickness.

What is balance? It's recalling our identity - bits of the heavenly, not separate from different creatures, yet one with them. Overlooking this Truth expedites infection, as per Barbara Ann Brennan, an outstanding profound healer and creator, who runs a school of healing in Long Island.

As per Diane Stein's Essential Reiki, certain feelings lead to specific sicknesses. What we feel moves toward becoming what we are made of, physically.

For instance, joint inflammation is brought about by a stickler frame of mind and analysis of self as well as other people, while disease originates from disdain, self centeredness and sadness. The issue of abundance weight is connected to sentiments of instability. Tumors are brought about by a refusal to heal.

"A lot of people say they want to get out of pain,

and I'm sure

that's true, but they aren't willing to make healing

a high priority.

They aren't willing to look inside to see the

source of their

pain in order to deal with it."

– Lindsay Wagner

The Reiki Principles

The Reiki standards improve otherworldly knowledge and can prompt change. Regardless of whether you haven't gotten an attunement, give them a shot and perceive how they feel to you. Anybody can rehearse them, regardless of whether they practice Reiki.

+ Just for today, I will give thanks for my many blessings.

+ Just for today, I will not worry.

✦ Just for today, I will not be angry.

✦ Just for today, I will do my work honestly.

✦ Just for today, I will be kind to my neighbor and every living thing.

Beside these standards, numerous things you want for your life can be rehearsed "only for now." See whether you can add anything to this rundown that you've been looking for in your life, out it an attempt today.

"I've experienced several different healing methodologies over the years - counseling, self-help seminars, and I've read a lot - but none of them

will work unless you really want to heal." –
Lindsay Wagner

When Reiki Doesn't Work

Here and there you'll see that your Reiki has no impact on your patient. Keep in mind that: you're just a channel for the vitality. For whatever length of time that you keep your fingers together (so the vitality doesn't escape through the holes) and contact the correct spots, the healing should work.

Be that as it may, at times the individual you're treating could obstruct the stream of vitality with his protection from recuperating. Truly, an individual may reveal to you that he's prepared for it, yet at an intuitive dimension, he isn't.

Some Reiki masters state that smoking and taking any type of medications can sloppy the Reiki channel, so driving a solid way of life will likewise make you an all the more dominant healer.

"The first wealth is health."

– Ralph Waldo Emerson

Two Important Premises of Reiki

One of the essential premises of Reiki is that it's not given free. You may ask why the all inclusive life vitality which is available in everything must be paid for. The appropriate response is that as indicated by the all inclusive law, there must be a trade of energy to keep up the concordance of the universe.

Additionally, this trade guarantees that there are no commitments on the beneficiary's side. There is agreement, not inbalance.

Another essential principle of Reiki is that it must be requested except if the beneficiary is in a condition where he can't ask for it.

You can, in any case, treat those you're straightforwardly in charge of without their asking for the healing. For example, it's alright to treat your relatives. It is, in any case, fitting to tell them your goals.

On account of a sluggish or missing individual, make sure to state rationally: "You are allowed to acknowledge or dismiss this healing as you will." This way you won't force your will upon the individual.

"To receive everything, one must open one's hands and give."

- Taisen Deshimaru

Conclusion

Eventually, Reiki gets through the healer, not from the healer. You are only a course for the vitality. To be best in your routine with regards to Reiki, discover a master with undeniable heredity. Likewise, watch out for your own wellbeing as it will improve you a healer.

Regardless of whether you have a Reiki attunement, the standards of Reiki can profit you. Only give it an attempt. You might be astonished at what you find out about yourself and your life!

Heal your mind, body and soul!

By Cice Rivera

www.ingramcontent.com/pod-product-compliance
Lightning Source LLC
Chambersburg PA
CBHW051124250726
48655CB00007B/2877